CHOLINE FOR BEGINNERS

Unlocking Cognitive Vitality, Harnessing Choline For Optimal Brain Health And Performance, Enhance Memory, Focus, And Overall Well-Being

Georgette Lockett

© [2023] [Georgette Lockett]

All rights reserved. No part of this publication may be reproduced, distributed, or transmitted in any form or by any means, including photocopying, recording, or other electronic or mechanical methods, without the prior written permission of the publisher, except in the case of brief quotations embodied in critical reviews and certain other noncommercial uses permitted by copyright law.

DISCLAIMER

The author of this book is not affiliated, associated, endorsed, sponsored, or approved by any company or individual. The views and opinions expressed in this book are solely those of the author and do not necessarily reflect the official policy or position of any entity.

The author hereby disclaims any relationship, collaboration, or partnership with any company or individual mentioned in this book. Any references to products, services, or individuals are provided for informational purposes only and should not be construed as an endorsement or recommendation.

Readers are advised to exercise their own judgment and discretion when applying the information provided in this book. The author shall not be held responsible for any actions taken by readers based on the content of this book.

This book is intended for general informational purposes only, and the author makes no representations or warranties of any kind, express or implied, about the completeness, accuracy, reliability, suitability, or availability of the information contained herein. Any reliance on the information in this book is at the reader's own risk.

The author reserves the right to update, change, or modify any information in this book without notice. It is the responsibility of the reader to verify any information before taking any actions based on the content of this book.

By reading this book, the reader acknowledges and agrees to the terms of this disclaimer.

INTRODUCTION

While choline is less well-known than certain other nutrients, it is critical to our general health and well-being. Here is a more in-depth explanation of its significance:

Understanding Choline: An Overview

Choline, which is often associated with B-complex vitamins, is an important nutrient that is necessary for a variety of physiological activities in the human body. It is necessary for brain development, cell structure, nerve function, and metabolism.

Importance Of Choline In Human Health

Choline is essential for brain function and cognition. It is a precursor of acetylcholine, a neurotransmitter that is essential for memory, mood modulation, and muscular function. It also helps with cell membrane shape and signaling.

Sources Of Choline In Diet

Although the body may create modest quantities of choline, it is mostly received from food. Choline-rich foods include eggs, liver, salmon, broccoli, and peanuts. However, many people do not eat enough, which may lead to a deficit.

Choline's Role In Bodily Functions

Choline has many functions in the body. It aids in lipid transport and metabolism, preventing fat formation in the liver. It also plays a role in methylation processes, which influence gene expression, cell repair, and neurotransmitter production.

Understanding choline's essential functions lays the groundwork for investigating its influence on numerous facets of human health.

CHAPTER 1

Choline Basics

Choline is an important ingredient that is required for many physiological functions in the human body. In this chapter, we will look at the fundamentals of choline, including its definition, chemical makeup, historical relevance, and nutritional categorization.

Defining Choline And Its Chemical Composition

Choline is a water-soluble component that is part of the B-vitamin complex but is not formally classified as a vitamin. It is distinguished from other B vitamins by the presence of a nitrogen-containing group in its chemical structure. Choline is crucial for the integrity and function of cells since it is a fundamental component of the structure of phospholipids.

Choline is a precursor for acetylcholine, a neurotransmitter that is essential for many nervous system activities such as muscular control, memory, and mood modulation. Choline is also involved in lipid metabolism, promoting fat transport and metabolism in the body.

Historical Perspective On Choline's Discovery

The discovery and acceptance of choline as a necessary nutrient has a long history. Choline was isolated in the early nineteenth century, and its significance in avoiding fatty liver was discovered in the mid-twentieth century. Scientists continued to uncover the numerous roles of choline as the study proceeded, emphasizing its relevance in cerebral development, liver health, and general well-being.

Choline's Classification In Nutrition

While choline is not formally classified as a vitamin, it is considered an important nutrient owing to its crucial functions in a variety of physiological processes. Although the body can generate some choline endogenously, food consumption is required to achieve total needs.

Because of its chemical composition and related effects, choline is sometimes paired alongside B vitamins. However, as scientific awareness of choline's activities and relevance has grown, so has its categorization.

In the next chapters, we will look at the many different elements of choline, such as its dietary sources, metabolism, and the consequences of choline deficit or insufficiency in the human body. Understanding the fundamentals of choline is critical for appreciating its relevance in sustaining health and avoiding possible deficits.

CHAPTER 2

Choline's Functions In The Body

Choline, an essential vitamin, is important for many biological processes and general health. Its importance extends to neurological development, brain health, liver function, cell structure, and other areas.

Choline's Role In Brain Development And Function

• **Neurodevelopment:** Choline is necessary for fetal development. It aids in the development of the brain and spinal cord, influencing neural tube closure and brain growth. Adequate choline consumption during pregnancy is linked to improved cognitive function in children.

• **Neurotransmitter Synthesis:** Choline regulates memory, mood, muscular control, and other cognitive processes as a precursor to acetylcholine, a neurotransmitter. It aids in the transmission of nerve impulses and signal transmission in the brain.

Choline's Impact On Cognitive Health

• **Memory and Learning:** Acetylcholine, a choline derivative, aids in memory formation and cognitive functions. Improved memory and learning capacities are connected to adequate choline levels in the body.

• **Concentration and attentiveness:** Choline's function in acetylcholine generation helps with mental concentration, attentiveness, and general cognitive performance.

Choline's Involvement In Nervous System Functions

• **Nerve Function:** Choline is required for the construction of cell membranes and the myelin sheath, which allows for effective nerve signaling and conductivity. This promotes normal nervous system function.

• **Mood Regulation:** Choline may regulate mood and emotional well-being by influencing neurotransmitter production, notably acetylcholine.

• **Cell Membrane Integrity:** Choline is a phospholipid component that is vital for cell membrane shape and integrity. It aids in the preservation of the structural integrity of cell membranes throughout the body.

• **Liver Health:** Choline has a role in lipid metabolism and fat transport from the liver. It aids in the prevention of fat formation in the liver and promotes overall liver health.

To summarize, choline is essential for brain development, cognitive function, nerve communication, and general cellular health due to its multiple activities.

Its effect goes beyond the brain to affect numerous physical systems, underscoring its significance in general well-being.

CHAPTER 3

Choline Deficiency And Health Implications

Symptoms And Signs Of Choline Deficiency

Choline is an essential vitamin, and a lack of it may appear in a variety of ways. Muscle damage, fatty liver, cognitive deficits, memory disorders, weariness, nerve damage, and even reproductive problems are possible symptoms. Some people may have higher amounts of homocysteine, a chemical associated with cardiovascular issues.

Health Conditions Linked To Choline Insufficiency

Choline deficiency may lead to liver illnesses such as non-alcoholic fatty liver disease (NAFLD) owing to its function in lipid metabolism, according to research.

Inadequate choline levels may be linked to cognitive diseases such as memory loss, decreased learning, and even neurological illnesses such as Alzheimer's disease. Furthermore, a lack of choline during pregnancy may affect embryonic brain development.

Impacts Of Choline Deficiency Across Different Age Groups

- **Infants and Children:** Low choline levels throughout early development may result in neural tube abnormalities and poor brain development.

- **Adolescents:** Deficiency throughout adolescence might impair cognitive processes, memory, and learning.

- **Adults:** Choline shortage may cause liver problems, decreased fat metabolism, and cognitive deterioration.

- **Older people:** Low choline levels may lead to cognitive impairment and neurological problems linked with aging.

It is critical to identify these possible consequences to prioritize proper choline consumption across all age groups.

The role of choline in different body activities emphasizes the need to maintain adequate amounts via diet or supplementation. Understanding the repercussions of choline insufficiency may assist in increasing awareness of choline's significance in general health and well-being.

CHAPTER 4

Dietary Sources Of Choline

Choline is an important vitamin that is required for many body activities. It is essential for brain development, neuron function, metabolism, and cellular structure. While the body may manufacture some choline, it is often required to get more via food or supplementation. Here's a detailed look at choline's dietary sources:

Natural Food Sources Rich In Choline

1. Egg yolks are one of the richest sources of choline. A big egg has around 147 mg of choline.

2. Liver: Particularly cow liver, which is high in choline. Over 300 mg of choline may be found in only 3 ounces.

3. Salmon, cod, and tilapia, in particular, contain moderate quantities of choline.

4. **Poultry:** Chicken and turkey are excellent suppliers, particularly the dark flesh and skin.

5. Milk, yogurt, and cheese all contain significant levels of choline.

6. Soybeans and peanuts are important sources of choline, giving a considerable quantity.

7. **Cruciferous Vegetables:** Broccoli, Brussels sprouts, and cauliflower have lower levels of choline.

8. **Quinoa:** Among grains, quinoa stands out as a choline source, but with a lesser amount than other sources.

9. Almonds, flaxseeds, and sunflower seeds all provide considerable quantities of choline.

Recommended Daily Intake Of Choline

• **Adults:** Adult males should consume 550 mg per day, while women should consume 425 mg per day. Pregnant women need around 450 mg per day, while lactating moms require 550 mg per day.

Challenges In Obtaining Adequate Choline From Diet Alone

Despite its significance, many individuals may not get enough choline owing to dietary choices, particularly if they avoid specific animal products or follow a limited diet. Vegetarians and vegans may have a more difficult time getting enough choline from plant-based sources.

Furthermore, cooking techniques, food processing, and storage all influence choline content. Choline levels in foods may be reduced by heat and extended cooking. Furthermore, processed grains often lack the choline present in whole grains.

Given these obstacles, supplementation or increased knowledge of choline-rich foods becomes critical to ensuring one's daily choline requirements for good health and well-being.

Understanding the dietary sources of choline assists in the preparation of balanced meals to guarantee optimal consumption. This information enables people to make intelligent food decisions based on their nutritional requirements.

CHAPTER 5

Choline And Pregnancy

Choline is essential for the development of the neurological system, especially during pregnancy. It is critical to emphasize its importance in maintaining healthy fetal growth and brain development while explaining its involvement in pregnancy.

Importance Of Choline During Pregnancy

Because of its role in brain development, especially the production of neural tube structures and cell membranes in the developing baby, choline is an essential vitamin throughout pregnancy. It functions as a precursor of acetylcholine, a neurotransmitter that is vital for brain transmission and cognitive function.

Choline's Role In Fetal Brain Development

According to research, enough choline consumption during pregnancy may have a good influence on a baby's brain development, perhaps improving cognitive function and memory later in life. It promotes neural tube closure and regulates brain cell development and structure. The significance of choline in neural stem cell proliferation and differentiation is critical for brain anatomical and functional development.

Recommended Choline Intake For Expecting Mothers

Pregnant women need more choline to support the growing baby. Adequate nutrition may assist both the mother and the baby throughout pregnancy. To assist fetal neurodevelopment, pregnant women should consume more vitamin D than non-pregnant people.

However, since choline is not frequently included in prenatal vitamins, many pregnant women do not reach the necessary consumption. As a result, dietary changes or supplementation may be required to guarantee appropriate levels. Choline-rich foods, such as eggs, lean meats, fish, and some plants like broccoli, may help considerably satisfy these needs.

Ensuring enough choline intake during pregnancy has the potential to improve cognitive outcomes for the kid and lower the likelihood of some neural tube abnormalities.

This chapter will dive into these topics, stressing the vital function of choline in pregnancy and the significance of attaining appropriate choline consumption levels for the optimum development of the developing baby.

CHAPTER 6

Choline And Cognitive Function

Impact Of Choline On Memory And Learning

Choline is important for cognitive function, especially memory and learning. It contributes to the establishment of brain connections linked with memory and learning processes as a precursor to acetylcholine, a neurotransmitter required for nerve transmission. According to research, choline availability may improve cognitive functions, possibly enhancing memory recall and information retention.

Choline's Influence On Age-Related Cognitive Decline

According to research, there may be a relationship between choline and age-related cognitive deterioration.

Adequate choline levels in the body may benefit cognitive health as people age. Choline deficiency has been linked to illnesses such as dementia and Alzheimer's disease, making it an important vitamin in fostering healthy brain aging.

Research And Studies On Choline's Cognitive Benefits

Numerous research have been conducted to evaluate the cognitive advantages of choline supplementation. Some studies have shown that those who consume enough choline have better cognitive function, attention span, and problem-solving ability. More study is being conducted to better understand the specific processes behind choline's benefits on cognitive functioning.

Choline's impact on brain development throughout the prenatal and early childhood periods is critical. Adequate choline consumption during pregnancy is thought to aid in a child's cognitive development and may even have long-term ramifications for brain health.

Regulation Of Neurotransmitters By Choline

Choline's involvement in the synthesis of acetylcholine, a neurotransmitter important in memory, attention, and muscular control, emphasizes its importance in brain function maintenance. It is also implicated in cognitive and general neurological health signaling pathways.

Choline Deficiency and Its Cognitive Consequences

Inadequate choline consumption may have cognitive consequences such as poor memory, decreased attention span, and diminished cognitive function. A shortage of choline may have a deleterious influence on brain development, particularly in fetuses and newborns, perhaps leading to cognitive impairments.

Understanding the function of choline in cognitive processes is critical for sustaining brain health throughout life, from early brain development to cognitive alterations associated with aging. Further research and study continue to provide light on the complex interaction between choline and cognitive function, perhaps providing new insights into cognitive health and techniques for cognitive improvement.

CHAPTER 7

Choline And Liver Health

The liver is a vital organ that is in charge of several metabolic activities such as detoxification, energy storage, and nutrition metabolism. Choline, while frequently overlooked, is essential for maintaining optimum liver function.

Choline's Role In Liver Function And Fat Metabolism

Choline serves as a precursor to phospholipids, which are essential components of cell membranes. It promotes the movement of lipids into and out of liver cells, reducing fat formation in the liver. Inadequate choline levels may cause fat metabolism to malfunction, resulting in fatty liver disease, which can proceed to more serious disorders such as non-alcoholic fatty liver disease (NAFLD) or non-alcoholic steatohepatitis (NASH).

Choline's Potential In Preventing Liver Diseases

According to research, choline insufficiency may lead to liver problems. Adequate choline intake, either via diet or supplementation, may aid in the prevention or treatment of liver disorders. Studies on choline's protective properties against liver damage induced by a variety of variables, including alcohol intake, pollutants, and some drugs, have shown encouraging findings.

Choline Supplementation For Liver Health

Individuals with liver disorders or those at risk of liver disease may benefit from choline supplements. However, before beginning any supplements, ask a healthcare practitioner since excessive choline consumption may have negative consequences and may interfere with certain drugs or health problems.

The Relationship Between Choline and Liver Function

Understanding the complex link between choline and liver function emphasizes the need to get enough choline. Incorporating choline-rich foods into one's diet, such as eggs, liver, fish, nuts, and cruciferous vegetables, benefits liver function. A balanced diet that fulfills recommended choline consumption levels also benefits overall liver health.

CHAPTER 8

Choline And Heart Health

Choline is essential for many biological activities, although it is often ignored in diet and health talks. This chapter will investigate the role of choline in heart health, including its influence on cardiovascular function and disease prevention.

Choline's Effects On Cardiovascular Health

Choline has gotten a lot of interest because of its ability to improve heart health. It is thought to reduce the risk of heart disease by influencing different cardiovascular indicators. According to research, choline is involved in the metabolism of homocysteine, an amino acid that has been linked to an increased risk of heart disease at high amounts.

Relationship Between Choline And Heart Disease

Choline's involvement in controlling homocysteine levels is critical since excessive homocysteine levels are linked to an increased risk of cardiovascular illnesses such as heart attacks and strokes. Choline aids in the conversion of homocysteine into other useful compounds, possibly decreasing the risk of heart disease.

Furthermore, choline's role in fat metabolism might indirectly benefit heart health. Adequate choline levels help in fat transport and metabolism in the liver, which may influence cholesterol levels and prevent fat buildup in the circulation.

Choline's Influence On Blood Lipid Levels

According to research, choline consumption may assist control of lipid profiles. Choline, along with other nutrients, seems to help keep cholesterol levels healthy. According to research, choline supplementation may reduce LDL cholesterol (commonly referred to as "bad" cholesterol) while boosting HDL cholesterol ("good" cholesterol). These effects are crucial because they contribute to a better lipid profile, which lowers the risk of atherosclerosis and cardiovascular disease.

Understanding the function of choline in cardiovascular health is critical for developing comprehensive methods to avoid heart disease. While studies on choline's influence on heart health are encouraging, further study is needed to explain the specific pathways and create optimum choline intake guidelines for heart health.

Individuals and healthcare providers can recognize the potential of choline in preventive strategies against heart-related conditions by emphasizing its importance in cardiovascular health, thereby advocating for a more balanced diet that includes choline-rich foods or supplements to promote overall heart health.

CHAPTER 9

Choline In Sports And Exercise

Choline's Impact On Athletic Performance

Choline, a necessary vitamin with several functions in the body, has received attention for its possible influence on athletic performance. Athletes and fitness enthusiasts are researching the advantages of choline supplementation to improve their training results.

Muscle Contraction And Neurotransmission

Choline's participation in neurotransmission is one of the most important features of its significance in exercise performance. Acetylcholine, a choline-derived neurotransmitter, is essential for communicating between neurons and muscles. During physical exercise, this neurotransmission is critical for muscle contraction and coordination.

Stamina And Endurance

Choline has been associated with increased endurance and stamina. According to research, maintaining enough choline levels may improve the body's capacity to sustain physical activity for longer periods. This may be especially advantageous for endurance athletes who participate in activities like running, cycling, or long-distance sports.

Cognitive And Motor Abilities

Aside from its effect on physical performance, choline has a significant impact on cognitive function. Improved cognitive function may help with motor abilities, decision-making, and general athletic coordination. Choline supplementation may be beneficial for athletes who participate in sports that demand accuracy and strategic thinking.

Choline's Role In Muscle Function And Recovery

Integrity of Muscle Cell Membrane

Choline is a component of phospholipids, which are important structural constituents of cell membranes. Muscle cell membrane integrity is critical for appropriate function and recovery. Choline's involvement in maintaining cell membrane health is especially important for athletes enduring severe exercise, as muscle cells are stressed and damaged.

Anti-Inflammatory Effects

Choline has anti-inflammatory effects, which may help to reduce inflammation caused by strenuous physical exercise. This anti-inflammatory impact may help athletes heal quicker, enabling them to continue training more effectively.

Synthesis of Muscle Proteins

Choline has been linked to muscle protein synthesis, which is essential for muscle development and repair. Maintaining optimum choline levels may help the efficacy of resistance training or muscular hypertrophy programs for athletes.

Choline Supplementation In Sports Nutrition

Choline Supplements in Different Forms

Choline supplements come in a variety of forms, including choline bitartrate and alpha-GPC. Understanding the distinctions and bioavailability of these forms is critical for athletes looking to add choline supplements to their diets.

Dosage & Administration

To maximize the effects of choline supplementation, the right dose and timing must be determined. Athletes can consider working with nutritionists or healthcare specialists to personalize choline supplements to their unique requirements, taking body weight, training intensity, and general health into consideration.

Considerations and Potential Risks

While choline supplementation may have some advantages, athletes should be mindful of the dangers and adverse effects. To avoid negative consequences, it is critical to balance choline consumption from food sources and supplementation.

To summarize, the function of choline in sports and exercise is an exciting field of study with intriguing implications for athletic performance. As our knowledge of choline's influence grows, athletes and fitness enthusiasts may include it in their training programs with the help of health specialists.

CHAPTER 10

Choline Supplements And Safety

Overview Of Choline Supplements

Choline supplements have gained popularity as a result of their possible health advantages. Understanding the nature of these supplements and their safety concerns is critical for anybody thinking about using them.

Choline supplements are available in a variety of forms, including choline bitartrate, choline chloride, and lecithin. They're often advertised for their alleged ability to improve brain health, liver function, and general well-being. The efficacy of these supplements, however, might vary depending on the chemical and formulation employed.

Safety Considerations And Possible Side Effects

Choline supplements are typically safe when used in the appropriate amounts. High dosages, on the other hand, might cause gastrointestinal upset, nausea, and fishy body odor. Individuals with specific health concerns, such as renal illness or trimethylaminuria, should see a healthcare practitioner before using choline supplements, since it may worsen these diseases.

Guidelines For Safe Choline Supplementation

It is critical for anyone contemplating choline supplementation to follow the prescribed dose parameters. The appropriate intake for choline varies by age and gender, with adult males recommended to eat around 550 mg per day and adult females recommended to consume approximately 425 mg per day. Pregnant and lactating women may need more choline. Before resorting to supplements, it's critical to get your choline from a well-balanced diet rich in eggs, liver, soy products, and other choline-containing foods.

It is important to understand that supplements are supposed to complement a healthy diet and lifestyle. They should not be used to substitute a nutrient-dense diet or as the only source of key elements such as choline.

Before beginning choline supplementation, as with any supplement, speak with a healthcare provider or a qualified dietician. This is particularly critical for those who have pre-existing health issues or are taking other drugs since interactions are possible.

Conclusion

Finally, research into choline has proven its important involvement in many facets of human health. Choline emerges as a diverse and vital vitamin, with effects ranging from brain development and cognitive health to liver function, cardiovascular health, and even sports performance. Understanding its value in pregnancy, where it aids in fetal brain development, emphasizes its significance in mother nutrition.

Choline insufficiency has been related to a variety of health issues, underlining the need to get enough via diet or supplementation. The identification of choline-rich foods and suggested daily consumption helps those seeking to maintain optimum choline levels with practical information.

Furthermore, the potential advantages of choline supplementation in certain health situations, such as liver disease or sports nutrition, bring up new possibilities for investigation and use. However, while introducing choline supplements into one's diet, it is critical to carefully evaluate safety requirements and any adverse effects.

As time goes on, the area of choline research promises to reveal new functions and uses for this crucial vitamin. More focused research on its influence on particular health disorders, the study of appropriate supplementation options, and continued attempts to promote awareness about choline's relevance in general well-being may be future avenues.

Choline is a complicated nutrient with far-reaching health and lifespan consequences. As research advances, including choline into dietary patterns and comprehending its potential for supplementation may contribute to a more holistic approach to health and well-being.

THE END